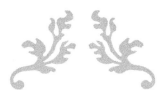

Low-Carb Cookbook

Discover How to Burn Stubborn Fat With Quick, Easy and
Flavorful Paleo Recipes | Over 50 Recipes from Breakfast to
Dinner

Albert Lee

Table of Contents

1. Cashew And Almond Butter

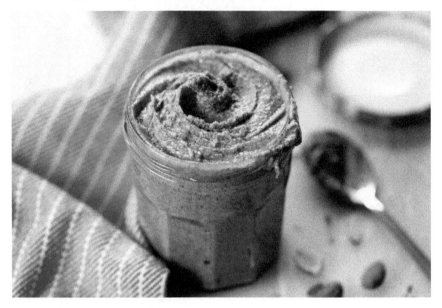

Serving: 1 and ½ cups

Prep Time: 5 minutes

Cook Time: Nil

Ingredients

- 1 cup almonds, blanched
- 1/3 cup cashew nuts
- 2 tablespoons coconut oil
- Salt as needed
- ½ teaspoon cinnamon

How To

1. Pre-heat your oven to 350 degree F

2. Bake almonds and cashews for 12 minutes

3. Let them cool

4. Transfer to food processor and add remaining ingredients

5. Add oil and keep blending until smooth

6. Serve and enjoy!

Nutrition (Per Serving)

- Calories: 205
- Fat: 19g
- Carbohydrates: g
- Protein: 2.8g

2. Crispy Walnut Crumbles

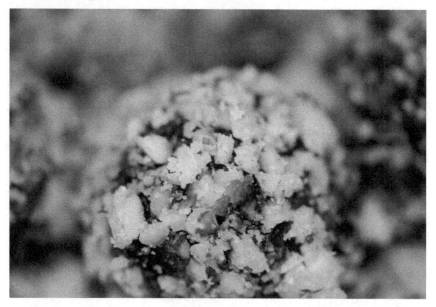

Serving: 10

Prep Time: 10 minutes

Cook Time: 8 minutes

Ingredients

- 6 ounces parmesan cheese, grated
- 2 tablespoons walnuts, chopped
- 1 tablespoons unsalted butter
- ½ tablespoon fresh thyme chopped

How To

1. Pre-heat your oven to 350 degree F

2. Take two large rimmed baking sheets and line with parchment

3. Add cheese, butter to food processor and blend

4. Add walnuts to the mix and pulse

5. Take a tablespoon and scoop mix onto baking sheet

6. Top with chopped thymes

7. Bake for 8 minutes, transfer to cooling rack

8. Let it cool for 30 minutes

9. Serve and enjoy!

Nutrition (Per Serving)

- Calories: 80
- Fat: 3g
- Carbohydrates: 7g
- Protein: 7g

3. Keto Kohlslaw

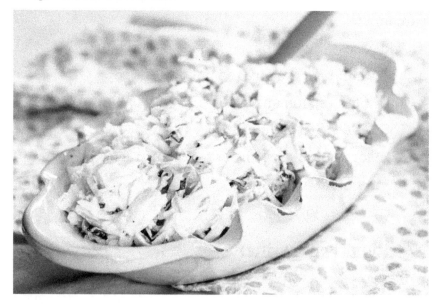

Serving: 4

Prep Time: 10 minutes

Cook Time: 0 minutes

Ingredients

- 1 pound kohlrabi, peeled and shredded
- Fresh parsley
- 1 cup mayonnaise (Keto-Friendly)
- Salt, to taste
- Ground black pepper, to taste

How To

1. Take a bowl and all the remaining ingredients

2. Mix it well until well combined

3. Adjust seasoning with salt and pepper

4. Serve and enjoy!

Nutrition (Per Serving)

- Calories: 392
- Fat: 40.4g
- Carbohydrates: 7.2g
- Protein: 6.2g

4. Stuffed Mushrooms

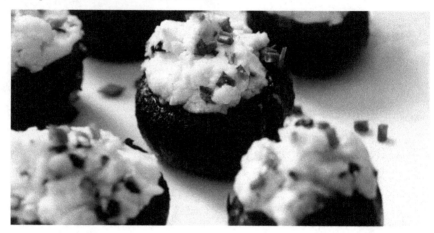

Serving: 4

Prep Time: 10 minutes

Cook Time: 15 minutes

Ingredients

- 4 Portobello mushroom
- 1 cup crumbled blue cheese
- 2 teaspoons extra virgin olive oil
- Salt, to taste
- Fresh thyme

How To

1. Preheat your oven to 350 degree Fahrenheit

2. Put out the stems from the mushrooms

3. Chop them into small pieces

4. Take a bowl and mix stem pieces with thyme, salt and blue cheese and mix well

5. Fill up mushroom with the prepared cheese

6. Top them with some oil

7. Take a baking sheet and place the mushrooms

8. Bake for 15 minutes to 20 minutes

9. Serve warm and enjoy!

Nutrition (Per Serving)

- Calories: 124
- Fat: 22.4g
- Carbohydrates: 5.4g
- Protein: 1.2g

5. Flax And Almond Crunchies

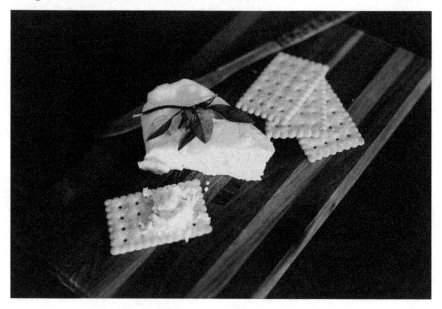

Serving: 20 Crackers

Prep Time: 15 minutes

Cook Time: 60 minutes

<u>Ingredients</u>

- ½ cup ground flax seeds
- ½ cup almond flour
- 1 tablespoon coconut flour
- 2 tablespoons shelled hemp seeds
- ¼ teaspoon sea salt, plus more to sprinkle on top
- 1 egg white
- 2 tablespoons unsalted butter, melted

How To

1. Pre-heat your oven to 300 degree F

2. Take a baking sheet and line it with parchment paper, keep the prepared sheet on the side

3. Add flax, coconut flour, almond, salt, hemp seed to a bowl and mix well

4. Add egg and melted butter, mix well

5. Transfer dough to sheet of parchment paper and cover with another sheet of paper

6. Roll out dough

7. Cut into crackers and bake for 60 minutes

8. Cool and serve!

Nutrition (Per Serving)

- Calories: 47
- Fat: 6g
- Carbohydrates: 1.2g
- Protein: 02g

6. Juicy Salmon Fat Bombs

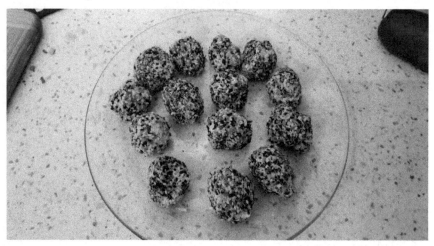

Serving: 12

Prep Time: 5 minutes

Cook Time: 10 minutes

Ingredients

- ½ cup goat cheese, at room temperature
- 2 teaspoons lemon juice, fresh
- ½ cup butter, at room temperature
- 2 ounces smoked salmon
- Black pepper to taste

How To

1. Place a parchment paper over baking sheet

2. Take a medium bowl and stir in goat cheese, smoked salmon, pepper, lemon juice together

3. Scoop it out into 12 mounds

4. Chill for 2-3 hours

5. Serve when needed and enjoy!

Nutrition (Per Serving)

- Calories:
- Fat: 18g
- Carbohydrates: 0g
- Protein: 8g

7. Roasted Herb Crackers

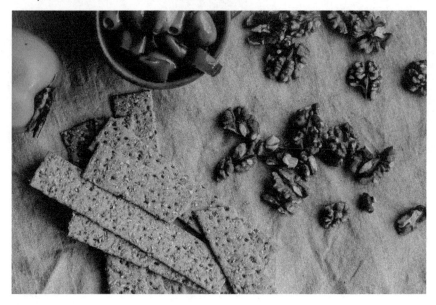

Serving: 75 Crackers

Prep Time: 10 minutes

Cook Time: 120 minutes

Ingredients

- ¼ cup avocado oil
- 10 celery sticks
- 1 sprig fresh rosemary, stem discarded
- 2 sprigs fresh thyme, stems discarded
- 2 tablespoons apple cider vinegar
- 1 teaspoon Himalayan salt
- 3 cups ground flax seeds

How To

1. Pre-heat your oven to 225 degree F

2. Line a baking sheet with parchment paper and keep it on the side

3. Add oil, herbs, celery, vinegar, salt to food processor and pulse until you have an even mixture

4. Add flax and puree

5. Let it sit for 2-3 minutes

6. Transfer batter to your prepared baking sheet and spread evenly, cut into cracker shapes

7. Bake for 60 minutes, flip and bake for 60 minutes more

8. Enjoy!

Nutrition (Per Serving)

- Calories: 34
- Fat: 5g
- Carbohydrates: 1g
- Protein: 1.3g

8. Crunchy Garlic Bread Stick

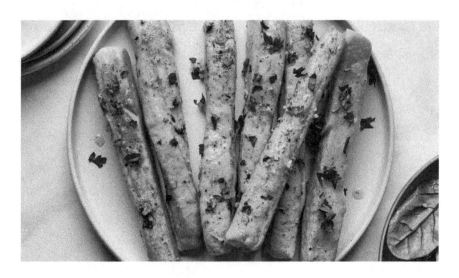

Serving: 8 bread sticks

Prep Time: 15 minutes

Cook Time: 15 minutes

Ingredients

- ¼ cup butter, softened
- 1 teaspoon garlic powder
- 2 cups almond flour
- ½ tablespoon baking powder
- 1 tablespoon Psyllium husk powder
- ¼ teaspoon salt
- 3 tablespoons butter, melted

- 1 egg
- ¼ cup boiling water

How To

1. Pre-heat your oven to 400-degree F

2. Line baking sheet with parchment paper and keep it on the side

3. Beat butter with garlic powder and keep it on the side

4. Add almond flour, baking powder, husk, salt in a bowl and mix in butter and egg, mix well

5. Pour boiling water in the mix and stir until you have a nice dough

6. Divide the dough into 8 balls and roll into breadsticks

7. Place on baking sheet and bake for 15 minutes

8. Brush each stick with garlic butter and bake for 5 minutes more

9. Serve and enjoy!

Nutrition (Per Serving)

- Calories: 259
- Fat: 24g
- Carbohydrates: 5g
- Protein: 7g

9. Magnificent Camembert Mushrooms

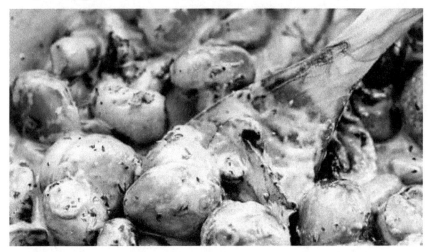

Serving: 4

Prep Time: 5 minutes

Cook Time: 13 minutes

Ingredients

- 2 tablespoons butter
- 4 ounces Camembert cheese, diced
- 2 teaspoons garlic, minced
- 1 pound button mushrooms, halved
- Black pepper to taste

How To

1. Place a skillet over medium high heat

2. Add butter and let it melt

3. Once the butter has melted, add garlic and Saute until translucent, should take 3 minutes

4. Add mushrooms and cook for 10 minutes

5. Season with pepper and serve

6. Enjoy!

<u>Nutrition (Per Serving)</u>

- Calories: 161
- Fat: 13g
- Carbohydrates: 3g
- Protein: 9g

10.   Golden Eggplant Fries

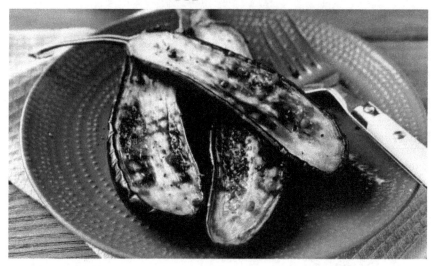

Serving: 8

Prep Time: 10 minutes

Cook Time: 15 minutes

Ingredients

- 2 eggs
- 2 cups almond flour
- 2 tablespoons coconut oil, spray
- 2 eggplant, peeled and cut thinly
- Salt and pepper

How To

1. Preheat your oven to 400 degree Fahrenheit

2. Take a bowl and mix with salt and black pepper in it

3. Take another bowl and beat eggs until frothy

4. Dip the eggplant pieces into eggs

5. Then coat them with flour mixture

6. Add another layer of flour and egg

7. Then, take a baking sheet and grease with coconut oil on top

8. Bake for about 15 minutes

9. Serve and enjoy!

Nutrition (Per Serving)

- Calories: 212
- Fat: 15.8g
- Carbohydrates: 12.1g
- Protein: 8.6g

11. Cheesy Mozzarella Sticks

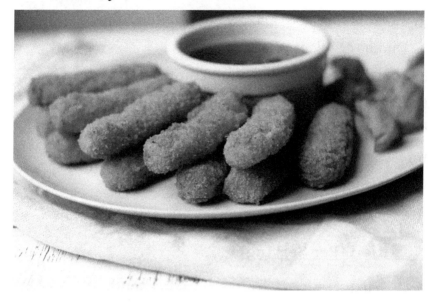

Serving: 8 bread sticks

Prep Time: 10 minutes

Cook Time: 20 minutes

Ingredients

- 2 cups shredded mozzarella cheese
- 2 tablespoons coconut flour
- 2 whole eggs
- 1 pinch of salt

Toppings

- ½ cup shredded parmesan cheese

- 1 tablespoons Italian seasoning
- ½ teaspoon garlic powder

How To

1. Pre-heat your oven to 350 degree F

2. Line a baking sheet with parchment paper

3. Take your food processor and add cheese, flour, eggs, salt and process

4. Scoop the mix onto your lined baking sheet and flatten to 1 inch thickness, forming a square

5. Bake for 15 minutes

6. Remove from oven and sprinkle parmesan cheese, Italian seasoning and garlic powder

7. Bake for 5 minutes

8. Remove from oven and let it cool

9. Serve and enjoy!

Nutrition (Per Serving)

- Calories: 225
- Fat: 19g
- Carbohydrates: 3g
- Protein: 12g

12.Salt And Rosemary Cracker

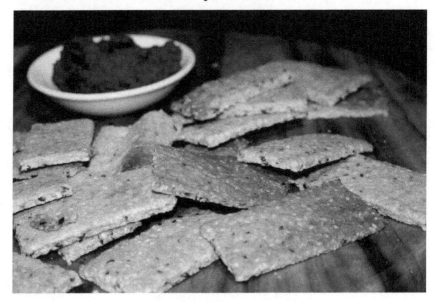

Serving: 36 Crackers

Prep Time: 10 minutes

Cook Time: 10-15 minutes

Ingredients

- 1 and ½ cups almond flour
- ½ teaspoon Celtic salt
- 1 egg, at room temp
- 2 tablespoons coconut oil
- ¼ teaspoon pepper
- 1 tablespoon rosemary, chopped

How To

1. Pre-heat oven to 350 degree F

2. Take a baking tray and line it with parchment paper

3. Take a bowl and add almond flour, salt and keep it on the side

4. Take another bowl and add coconut oil, pepper, rosemary

5. Add almond mix to the bowl

6. Mix well until you have an even dough

7. Transfer dough to a piece of parchment paper, cover with another parchment paper piece and roll it out into a thin layer

8. Cut into crackers, arrange them on prepped baking sheet

9. Bake for 10-15 minutes

10. Let them cool

11. Serve and enjoy!

Nutrition (Per Serving)

- Calories: 66
- Fat: 6g
- Carbohydrates: 1.4g
- Protein: 3g

13. Premium Goat Cheese Salad

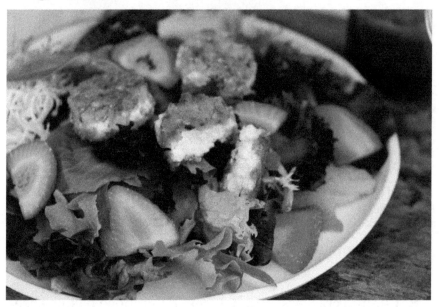

Serving: 2

Prep Time: 4 minutes

Cook Time: 10 minutes

<u>Ingredients</u>

- 1 and ½ cups Hard Goat cheese, grated
- 4 cups spinach, fresh
- 4 strawberries, garnish
- ½ cup flaked almonds, toasted
- 4 tablespoons Raspberry vinaigrette, check for Keto-Friendliness

How To

1. Pre-heat your oven to 400 degree F

2. Line a baking sheet using parchment paper, cut the parchment paper in half

3. Grate goat cheese onto each half

4. Form two circles using the grated cheese

5. Bake for 10 minutes

6. Transfer to a bowl and let it cool in the bowl shape

7. Peel the cheese off

8. Add remaining ingredients into the cheese and toss well

9. Serve immediately and enjoy!

Nutrition (Per Serving)

- Calories: 645
- Fat: 53g
- Carbohydrates: 6g
- Protein: 33g

14. Grilled Avocado And Melted Cheese

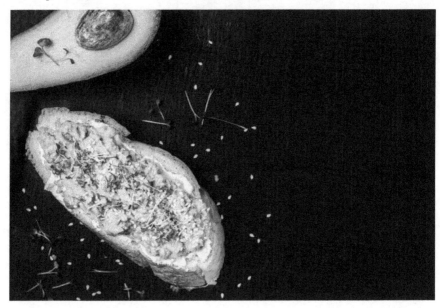

Serving: 6

Prep Time: 5 minutes

Cook Time: 4 minutes

Ingredients

- 1 whole avocado
- 1 tablespoon chipotle sauce
- 1 tablespoon lime juice
- ¼ cup parmesan cheese
- Salt and pepper to taste

How To

1. Prepare avocado by slicing half lengthwise, and discard seed

2. Gently prick skin of avocado with fork

3. Set your avocado halves, skin down on small baking sheet, lined with aluminum foil

4. Top with sauce and drizzle lime juice

5. Season with salt and pepper

6. Sprinkle half parmesan cheese in each cavity, set your broiler to high for 2 minutes

7. Add rest of the cheese and return to your broiler until cheese melts and avocado slightly browns

8. Serve hot and enjoy!

Nutrition (Per Serving)

- Calories: 459
- Fat: 41g
- Carbohydrates: 15g
- Protein: 7g

15. Mozzarella And Bacon Bites

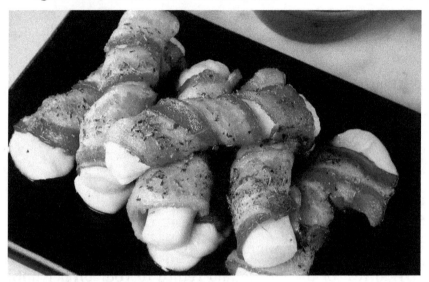

Serving: 4

Prep Time: 10 minutes

Cook Time: 5 minutes

Ingredients

- 8 bacon strips
- 4 mozarella string cheese pieces
- Olive oil, as needed

How To

1. Take a heavy duty skillet and place it over medium heat

2. Add 2 inch of oil, let it heat up to 350 degree F (check using thermometer)

3. Cut the string cheese to 8 pieces

4. Wrap each piece string cheese with a strip of bacon and secure using toothpick

5. Cook the sticks in hot oil for 2 minutes until the bacons are browned

6. Transfer to serving platter and drain with kitchen towel

7. Serve!

Nutrition (Per Serving)

- Calories: 278
- Fat: 15g
- Carbohydrates: 3g
- Protein: 32g

16.Brazilian Butter Macadamia

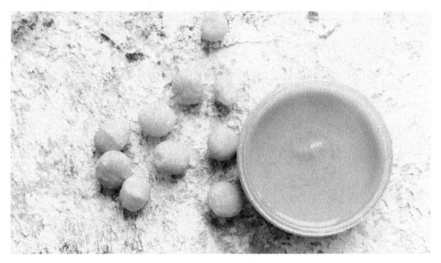

Serving: 1 and ½ cups

Prep Time: 5 minutes

Cook Time: Nil

Ingredients

- 2 tablespoons chives, fresh and chopped
- 1 tablespoon lemon juice, fresh
- ¼ cup Keto-Friendly mayonnaise
- ½ avocado, large
- 3 egg yolks, large and cooked

How To

1. Add listed ingredients to a food processor and blend until smooth

2. Scrap the sides and transfer to a mason jar

3. Serve when needed!

Nutrition (Per Serving)

- Calories: 225
- Fat: 23g
- Carbohydrates: 1.7g
- Protein: 2.8g

17. Tasty Roasted Broccoli

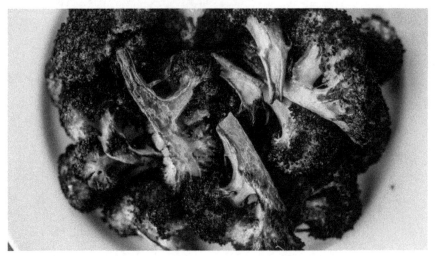

Serving: 4

Prep Time: 5 minutes

Cook Time: 20 minutes

Ingredients

- 4 cups broccoli florets
- 1 tablespoon olive oil
- Salt and pepper to taste

How To

1. Pre-heat your oven to 400 degree F

2. Add broccoli in a zip bag alongside oil and shake until coated

3. Add seasoning and shake again

41

4. Spread broccoli out on baking sheet, bake for 20 minutes

5. Let it cool and serve

6. Enjoy!

Nutrition (Per Serving)

- Calories: 62
- Fat: 4g
- Carbohydrates: 4g
- Protein: 4g

18.Spicy Pimento Cheese Dip

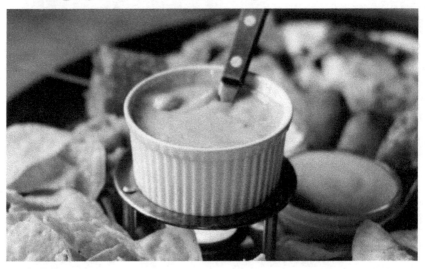

Serving: 10

Prep Time: 5 minutes

Cook Time: 5 minutes

Ingredients

- 1 brick cream cheese
- 10 cherry peppers, chopped
- 1 and ½ cups cheddar cheese, shredded
- 1 tablespoon garlic, minced
- Black pepper to taste

How To

1. Heat up garlic in a pan over medium heat

2. Drop cream cheese and let it soft, stir consistently

3. Mix in cheddar, add chopped peppers

4. Stir and enjoy with your desired dippers!

Nutrition (Per Serving)

- Calories: 259
- Fat: 24g
- Carbohydrates: 4g
- Protein: 16g

19. Bacon Smoky Doodles

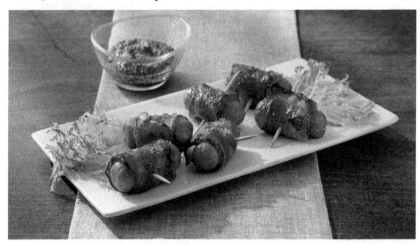

Serving: 4

Prep Time: 5 minutes

Cook Time: 25 minutes

Ingredients

- 24 little Smokies (Sausages)
- 3 tablespoons BBQ sauce, check for Keto Friendliness
- Salt and pepper to taste
- 6 slices bacon

How To

1. Pre-heat your oven to 375 degree F

2. Cut bacon into quarter pieces

3. Put sausage on each one and roll bacon over them, use a toothpick to secure it properly

4. Bake for 25 minutes and baste with BBQ sauce

5. Bake for 10 minutes more

6. Serve and enjoy!

<u>Nutrition (Per Serving)</u>

- Calories: 247
- Fat: 18g
- Carbohydrates: 2g
- Protein: 14g

20.   Tantalizing Butter Beans

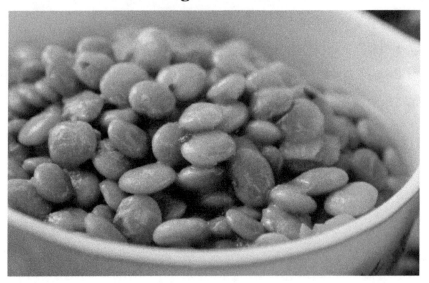

Serving: 4

Prep Time: 5 minutes

Cook Time: 12 minutes

Ingredients

- 2 garlic cloves, minced
- Red pepper flakes to taste
- Salt to taste
- 2 tablespoons clarified butter
- 4 cups green beans, trimmed

How To

1. Bring a pot of salted water to boil

2. Once the water starts to boil, add beans and cook for 3 minutes

3. Take a bowl of ice water and drain beans, plunge them in the ice water

4. Once cooled, keep them on the side

5. Take a medium skillet and place it over medium heat, add ghee and melt

6. Add red pepper, salt, garlic

7. Cook for 1 minute

8. Add beans and toss until coated well, cook for 3 minutes

9. Serve and enjoy!

<u>Nutrition (Per Serving)</u>

- Calories: 93
- Fat: 8g
- Carbohydrates: 4g
- Protein: 2g

21. Walnuts And Asparagus Delight

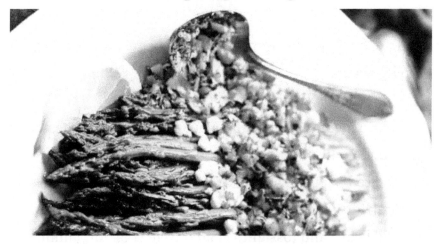

Serving: 4

Prep Time: 5 minutes

Cook Time: 5 minutes

Ingredients

- 1 and ½ tablespoons olive oil
- ¾ pound asparagus, trimmed
- ¼ cup walnuts, chopped
- Salt and pepper to taste

How To

1. Place a skillet over medium heat add olive oil and let it heat up

2. Add asparagus, Saute for 5 minutes until browned

3. Season with salt and pepper

4. Remove heat

5. Add walnuts and toss

6. Serve warm!

<u>Nutrition (Per Serving)</u>

- Calories: 124
- Fat: 12g
- Carbohydrates: 2g
- Protein: 3g

22.   Spicy Chili Crackers

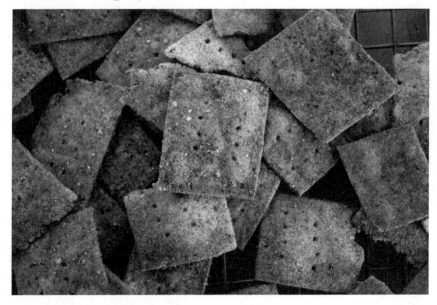

Serving: 30 crackers

Prep Time: 15 minutes

Cook Time: 60 minutes

Ingredients

- ¾ cup almond flour
- ¼ cup coconut four
- ¼ cup coconut flour
- ½ teaspoon paprika
- ½ teaspoon cumin
- 1 and ½ teaspoons chili pepper spice
- 1 teaspoon onion powder

- ½ teaspoon salt
- 1 whole egg
- ¼ cup unsalted butter

How To

1. Pre-heat your oven to 350 degree F

2. Take a baking sheet and line it up with parchment paper, keep it on the side

3. Add listed ingredients to food processor and process until you have a nice and firm dough

4. Divide dough into two equal parts

5. Place one ball on sheet of parchment paper and cover it with another paper

6. Roll it out

7. Cut into crackers and do the same with the other ball

8. Transfer dough to your prepared baking dish and bake for 8-10 minutes

9. Remove from oven and serve

10. Enjoy!

Nutrition (Per Serving)

- Calories: 49
- Fat: 4.1g
- Carbohydrates: 3g
- Protein: 1.6g

23.   Faux Mac And Cheese

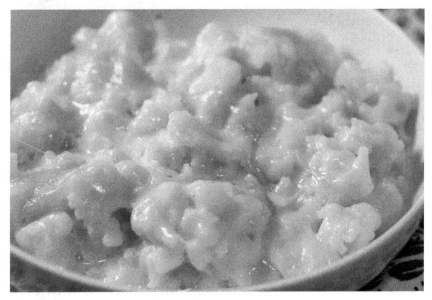

Serving: 4

Prep Time: 15 minutes

Cook Time: 45 minutes

Ingredients

- 5 cups cauliflower florets
- Salt and pepper to taste
- 1 cup coconut milk
- ½ cup vegetable broth
- 2 tablespoon coconut flour, sifted
- 1 organic egg, beaten
- 2 cups cheddar cheese

How To

1. Pre-heat your oven to 350 degree F

2. Season florets with salt and steam until firm

3. Place florets in greased oven proof dish

4. Heat coconut milk over medium heat in a skillet, make sure to season the oil with salt and pepper

5. Stir in broth and add coconut flour to the mix, stir

6. Cook until the sauce begins to bubble

7. Remove heat and add beaten egg

8. Pour the thick sauce over cauliflower and mix in cheese

9. Bake for 30-45 minutes

10. Serve and enjoy!

Nutrition (Per Serving)

- Calories: 229
- Fat: 14g
- Carbohydrates: 9g
- Protein: 15g

24.   Hearty Roasted Cauliflower

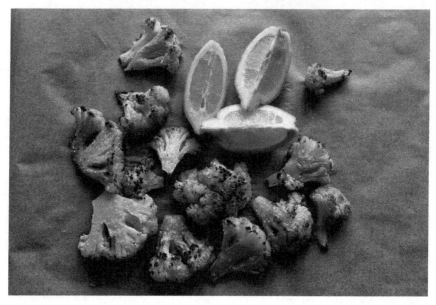

Serving: 8

Prep Time: 5 minutes

Cook Time: 30 minutes

Ingredients

- 1 large cauliflower head
- 2 tablespoons melted coconut oil
- 2 tablespoons fresh thyme
- 1 teaspoon Celtic sea salt
- 1 teaspoon fresh ground pepper
- 1 head roasted garlic
- 8 ounces burrata cheese, for garnish

- 2 tablespoons fresh thyme for garnish

How To

1. Pre-heat your oven to 425 degree F
2. Rinse cauliflower and trim, core and sliced
3. Lay cauliflower evenly on rimmed baking tray
4. Drizzle coconut oil evenly over cauliflower, sprinkle thyme leaves
5. Season with pinch of salt and pepper
6. Squeeze roasted garlic
7. Roast cauliflower until slightly caramelize for about 30 minutes, making sure to turn once
8. Garnish with fresh thyme leaves and burbata
9. Enjoy!

Nutrition (Per Serving)

- Calories: 129
- Fat: 11g
- Carbohydrates: 6g
- Protein: 7g

25.   Sausage And Shrimp Skewers

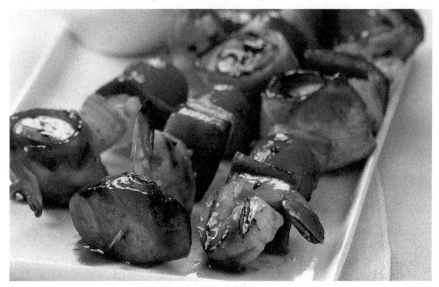

Serving: 6

Prep Time: 20 minutes

Cook Time: 10 minutes

Ingredients

- 3 large smoked sausages cut into 30-35 slices in total
- 2 medium-sized zucchinis, cut into 35-40 slices
- 40 shrimps, peeled with tail on
- 1 batch of low carb barbeque sauce

How To

1. Take each skewer and thread 2 pieces of shrimp, two zucchini, and two sausages (one ingredient, then another to make a pattern).

2. Brush the barbeque sauce over the shrimp and zucchini and cook over a grill pan for 3-4 minutes on each side.

3. Serve optionally with chopped lettuce and some extra barbeque sauce

Nutrition (Per Serving)

- Calories: 178
- Fat: 12g
- Carbohydrates: 3g
- Protein: 12g

26.   Fancy Grilled Halloumi Bruschetta

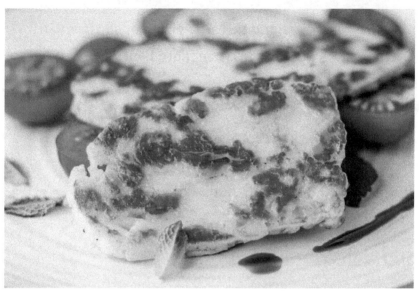

Serving: 4

Prep Time: 10 minutes

Cook Time: 10 minutes

<u>Ingredients</u>

- 2 medium tomatoes, chopped
- 2 packages of halloumi cheese (Cyprus grilling cheese), cut into 1 inch thick slices lengthwise
- 2 tbsp of olive oil
- 1 tbsp of chopped fresh basil leaves, chopped

How To

1. In a bowl, combine the tomatoes with the basil and 1 tbsp of olive oil.

2. Heat the remaining tsp of olive oil in a grilling pan and add the halloumi cheese slices to grill for around 2 minutes on each side.

3. Serve the halloumi slices with the tomato mixture on top, as if you are making a bruschetta

Nutrition (Per Serving)

- Calories: 134
- Fat: 12.4g
- Carbohydrates: 1g
- Protein: 7g

27.   Broccoli And Dill Salad

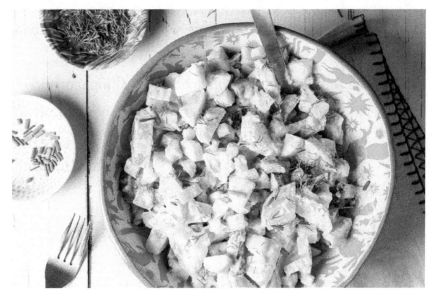

Serving: 4

Prep Time: 10 minutes

Cook Time: 5 minutes

<u>Ingredients</u>

- 1 pound (454 g) broccoli, cut into florets and stems
- 3/4 cup fresh dill
- 1 cup keto-friendly mayonnaise
- 1l2 teaspoon ground pepper
- 1l2 teaspoon salt

How To

1. Boil the broccoli florets and stems in a pot of lightly salted water for about 5 minutes, or until it becomes fork-tender but firm and greenish.

2. Using a colander, drain the broccoli then put it in a medium bowl. Add the fresh dill, mayonnaise and mix gently. Lightly season with pepper and salt before serving.

Nutrition (Per Serving)

- Calories: 406
- Fat: 42g
- Carbohydrates: 5g
- Protein: 5g

28.   Cheddar Biscuits

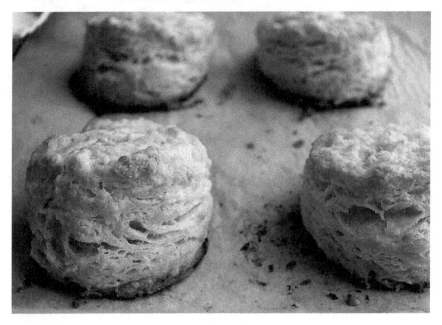

Serving: 4

Prep Time: 10 minutes

Cook Time: 30 minutes

Ingredients

- 2 1/2 cups almond flour
- 2 tsp baking powder
- 2 eggs beaten
- 3 tbsp melted butter
- 3/4 cup grated cheddar cheese

How To

1. Preheat oven to 350 F; line a baking sheet with parchment paper. In a bowl, mix flour, baking powder, and eggs until smooth.

2. Whisk in the melted butter and cheddar cheese until well combined.

3. Mold 12 balls out of the mixture and arrange them on the sheet at 2-inch intervals.

4. Bake for 25 minutes until golden brown. Remove, let cool and serve

Nutrition (Per Serving)

- Calories: 355
- Fat: 28g
- Carbohydrates: 1.14g
- Protein: 21g

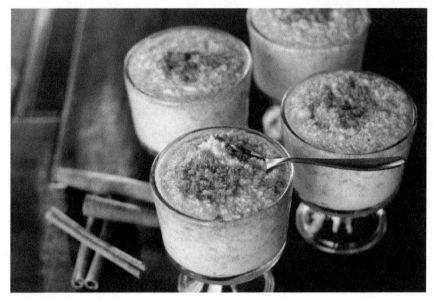

Serving: 4

Prep Time: 15 minutes

Cook Time: Nil

Ingredients

- 1 1/4 cups coconut cream
- 1 tsp vanilla extract
- 1 tsp cinnamon powder
- 1 cup mashed tofu
- 2 oz fresh strawberries

How To

1. Pour coconut cream into a bowl and whisk until a soft peak forms. Mix in vanilla and cinnamon.

2. Lightly fold in tofu and refrigerate for 10-15 minutes to set. Spoon into Serves glasses, top with the strawberries, and serve

Nutrition (Per Serving)

- Calories: 225
- Fat: 20g
- Carbohydrates: 3g
- Protein: 6g

30. Almond Flour English Cake

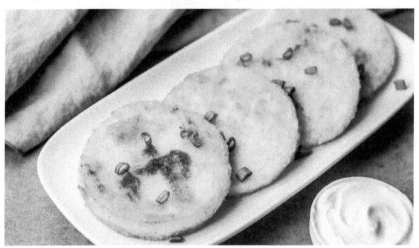

Serving: 4

Prep Time: 10 minutes

Cook Time: 10-15 minutes

Ingredients

- 2 tbsp flax seed powder + 6 tbsp water
- 2 tbsp almond flour
- 1/2 tsp baking powder
- 1 pinch salt
- 3 tbsp vegan butter

How To

1. In a bowl, mix flax seed with water until evenly combined, and leave to soak for 5 minutes.

2. In another bowl, combine almond flour, baking powder, and salt. Then, pour in the flax egg and whisk again.

3. Let the batter sit for 5 minutes to set. Melt the vegan butter in a frying pan over medium heat, and add the mixture in four dollops.

4. Fry until golden brown on one side, then flip the bread with a spatula and fry further until golden brown.

5. Serve with tea

<u>Nutrition (Per Serving)</u>

- Calories: 161
- Fat: 13g
- Carbohydrates: 2g
- Protein: 7g

31. Bacon And Avocado Fat Bombs

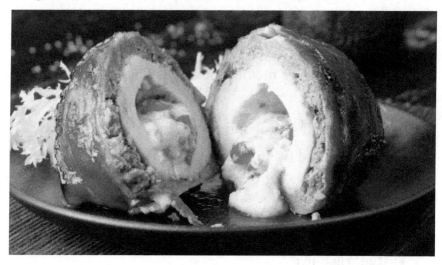

Serving: 4

Prep Time: 10 minutes

Cook Time: 50 minutes

Ingredients

- 1 avocado, halved, pitted
- 4 slices of bacon
- 2 tbsp grated parmesan cheese

How To

1. Turn on the oven and broiler and let it preheat. Meanwhile, prepare the avocado and for that, cut it in half, then remove its pit, and then peel the skin.

2. Evenly cover one half of the avocado with cheese, replace with the other half of avocado and then wrap avocado with bacon slices.

3. Take a baking sheet, line it with aluminum foil, place wrapped avocado on it, and broil for 5 minutes per side, flipping carefully with tong halfway.

4. When done, cut each avocado in half crosswise and serve

Nutrition (Per Serving)

- Calories: 336
- Fat: 15g
- Carbohydrates: 2.3g
- Protein: 0.5g

32. Green Olives With Deviled Eggs

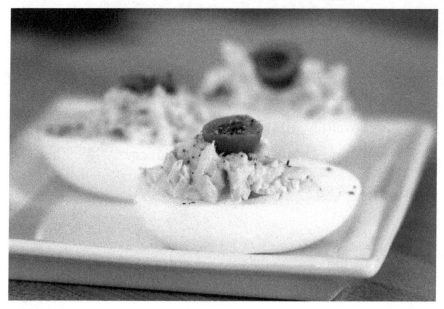

Serving: 2

Prep Time: 10 minutes

Cook Time: Nil

Ingredients

- 2 eggs, boiled
- 1 tbsp chopped green olives
- 1/4 tsp paprika
- 2 tbsp mayonnaise
- 1 tbsp cream cheese, softened

How To

1. Peel the boiled eggs, then slice in half lengthwise and transfer egg yolks to a medium bowl by using a spoon.

2. Mash the egg yolk, add remaining ingredients and stir until well combined.

3. Spoon the egg yolk mixture into egg whites and then serve.

Nutrition (Per Serving)

- Calories: 209
- Fat: 8g
- Carbohydrates: 0.2g
- Protein: 1.4g

33.   Spinach And Bacon Salad

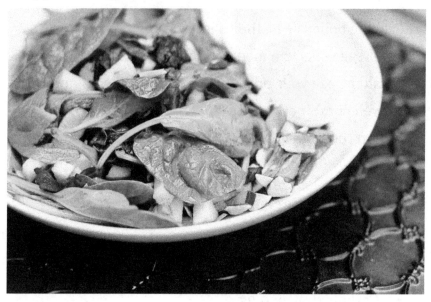

Serving: 2

Prep Time: 10 minutes

Cook Time: 5 minutes

Ingredients

- 4 oz spinach
- 4 sliced of bacon, chopped
- 2 eggs, boiled, sliced
- ¹/a cup mayonnaise

How To

1. Take a skillet pan, place it over medium heat, add bacon, and cook for 5 minutes until browned.

2. Meanwhile, take a salad bowl, add spinach

3. in it, top with bacon and eggs and drizzle with mayonnaise.

4. Toss until well mixed and then serve.

Nutrition (Per Serving)

- Calories: 181
- Fat: 8g
- Carbohydrates: 0.3g
- Protein: 0.2g

34.   Cool Bacon And Cheese Rolls

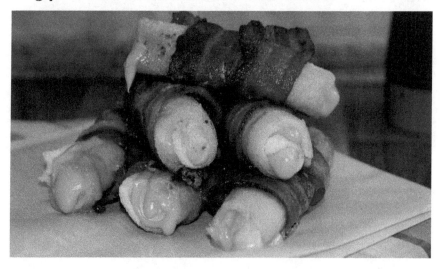

Serving: 4

Prep Time: 10 minutes

Cook Time: 50 minutes

Ingredients

- 2 oz mozzarella cheese, sliced, full-fat
- 4 slices of bacon

How To

1. Take a skillet pan, place it over medium heat and when hot, add bacon slices and cook for 3 minutes per side until crisp.
2. When done, transfer bacon to the cutting board, cool for 5 minutes, and then chop.

3. Cut cheese into thin slices, top with chopped bacon, and then roll the cheese.

4. Serve.

Nutrition (Per Serving)

- Calories: 165
- Fat: 12g
- Carbohydrates: 0.8g
- Protein: 0.8g

35.   Roasted Brussels And Bacon

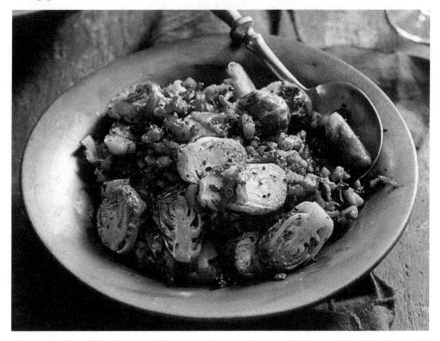

Serving: 4

Prep Time: 10 minutes

Cook Time: 35-40 minutes

Ingredients

- 24 oz brussels sprouts
- ¹/4 cup fish sauce
- ¹/4 cup bacon grease
- 6 strips bacon Pepper to taste

How To

1. De-stem and quarter the brussels sprouts.

2. Mix them with the bacon grease and fish sauce.

3. Slice the bacon into small strips and cook.

4. Add the bacon and pepper to the sprouts.

5. Spread onto a greased pan and cook at 450°F/230°C for 35 minutes.

6. Stir every 5 minutes or so.

7. Broil for a few more minutes and serve.

Nutrition (Per Serving)

- Calories: 130
- Fat: 9g
- Carbohydrates: 5g
- Protein: 7g

36.   Parmesan Garlic Cauliflower

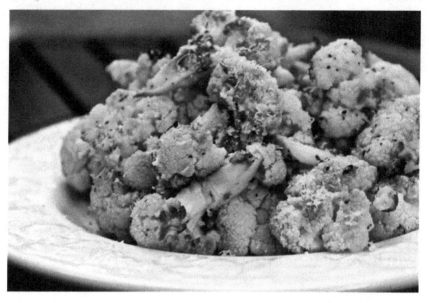

Serving: 4

Prep Time: 10 minutes

Cook Time: 50 minutes

Ingredients

- 3/4 cup cauliflower florets 2 tbsp butter
- 1 clove garlic, sliced thinly
- 2 tbsp shredded parmesan 1 pinch of salt

How To

1. Preheat your oven to 350°F/175°C.

2. On low heat, melt the butter with the garlic for 5-10 minutes.

3. Strain the garlic in a sieve.

4. Add the cauliflower, parmesan, and salt.

5. Bake for 20 minutes or until golden.

6. Serve and enjoy once done!

<u>Nutrition (Per Serving)</u>

- Calories: 180
- Fat: 18g
- Carbohydrates: 6g
- Protein: 7g

37.   Flaxy Cheese Chips

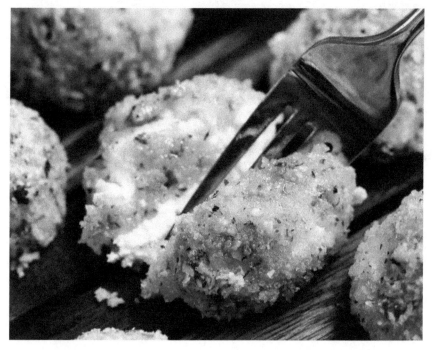

Serving: 4

Prep Time: 10 minutes

Cook Time: 10-15 minutes

Ingredients

- 1 1/2 cup cheddar cheese
- 4 tbsp ground flaxseed meal
- Seasonings of your choice

How To

1. Preheat your oven to 425°F/220°C.

2. Spoon 2 tablespoons of cheddar cheese into a mound onto a non-stick pad.

3. Spread out a pinch of flax seed on each chip.

4. Season and bake for 10-15 minutes.

5. Serve and enjoy!

Nutrition (Per Serving)

- Calories: 130
- Fat: 8g
- Carbohydrates: 1g
- Protein: 5g

38.   Handy Baked Tortillas

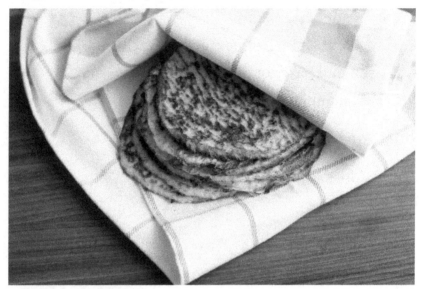

Serving: 4

Prep Time: 10 minutes

Cook Time: 20-30 minutes

<u>Ingredients</u>

- 1 large head of cauliflower, divided into florets. 4 large eggs
- 2 garlic cloves (minced)
- 1 1/2 tsp herbs (whatever your favorite is - basil, oregano, thyme)
- 1/2 tsp salt

How To

1. Preheat your oven to 375°F/190°C.
2. Put parchment paper on two baking sheets.
3. In a food processor, break down the cauliflower into rice.
4. Add 1/4 cup water and the riced cauliflower to a saucepan.
5. Cook on medium-high heat until tender for 10 minutes. Drain.
6. Dry with a clean kitchen towel.
7. Mix the cauliflower, eggs, garlic, herbs, and salt.
8. Make 4 thin circles on the parchment paper.
9. Bake for 20 minutes, until dry.
10. Serve and enjoy!

Nutrition (Per Serving)

- Calories: 90
- Fat: 6g
- Carbohydrates: 4g
- Protein: 3g

39.   Fine Jarlsberg Omelet

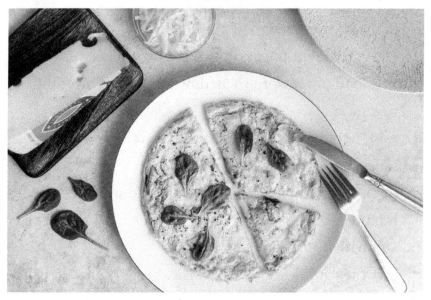

Serving: 4

Prep Time: 10 minutes

Cook Time: 5 minutes

<u>Ingredients</u>

- 4 medium mushrooms, sliced, 2 oz
- 1 green onion, sliced
- 2 eggs, beaten
- 1 oz Jarlsberg or Swiss cheese, shredded 1 oz ham, diced

How To

1. In a skillet, cook the mushrooms and green onion until tender.
2. Add the eggs and mix well.
3. Sprinkle with salt and top with the mushroom mixture, cheese, and ham.
4. When the egg is set, fold the plain side of the omelet on the filled side.
5. Turn off the heat and let it stand until the cheese has melted.
6. Serve!

Nutrition (Per Serving)

- Calories: 525
- Fat: 37g
- Carbohydrates: 15g
- Protein: 40g

40.   Asparagus And Baked Pork

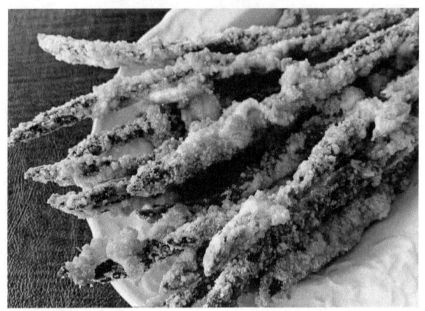

Serving: 4

Prep Time: 10 minutes

Cook Time: 20 minutes

Ingredients

- 1 pound (454 g) asparagus, tough ends removed
- ½ *cup* roughly ground pork rinds
- 1 cup ranch dressing Pinch of sea salt

How To

1. Arrange the asparagus spears in a casserole dish. Spread the pork rinds and ranch dressing over the asparagus, then season with sea salt.

2. Place the casserole dish in the preheated oven and bake for 18 minutes or until lightly browned.

3. Transfer them onto a platter and serve warm.

Nutrition (Per Serving)

- Calories: 303
- Fat: 7g
- Carbohydrates:298g
- Protein: 8g

41.Spicy Fired Up Jalapeno Poppers

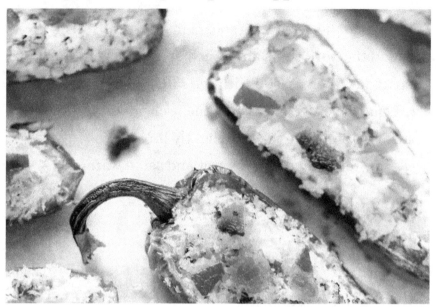

Serving: 4

Prep Time: 10 minutes

Cook Time: 30 minutes

Ingredients

- 5 oz cream cheese
- ¹/4 cup mozzarella cheese
- 8 medium jalapeno peppers
- ¹/2 tsp Mrs. Dash Table Blend
- 8 slices bacon

How To

1. Preheat your oven to 400°F/200°C.
2. Cut the jalapenos in half.
3. Use a spoon to scrape out the insides of the peppers.
4. In a bowl, add together the cream cheese, mozzarella cheese, and spices of your choice.
5. Pack the cream cheese mixture into the jalapenos and place the peppers on top.
6. Wrap each pepper in 1 slice of bacon, starting from the bottom and working up.
7. Bake for 30 minutes. Broil for an additional 3 minutes.
8. Serve!

Nutrition (Per Serving)

- Calories: 550
- Fat: 12g
- Carbohydrates: 5g
- Protein: 5g

42.   Bacon And Chicken Patties

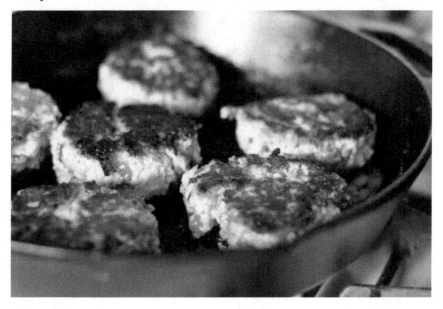

Serving: 4

Prep Time: 10 minutes

Cook Time: 10-15 minutes

Ingredients

- 12 oz can chicken breast
- 4 slices bacon
- 1/4 cup parmesan cheese
- 1 large egg
- 3 tbsp keto coconut flour

How To

1. Cook the bacon until crispy.
2. Chop the chicken and bacon together in a food processor until fine.
3. Add in the parmesan, egg, coconut flour, and mix.
4. Make the patties by hand and fry on medium heat in a pan with some oil.
5. Once browned, flip over, continue cooking, and lie them to drain.
6. Serve!

Nutrition (Per Serving)

- Calories: 420
- Fat: 22g
- Carbohydrates: 4g
- Protein: 37g

43.   Juicy Grilled Ham And Cheese

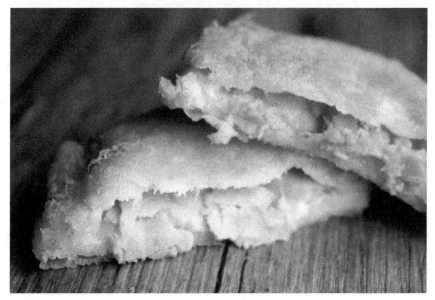

Serving: 4

Prep Time: 10 minutes

Cook Time: 20-30 minutes

<u>Ingredients</u>

- 3 low-carb keto buns
- 4 slices medium-cut deli ham 1 tbsp salted butter
- 3 slices cheddar cheese 1/2 cup almond flour
- 1 tsp. baking powder
- 2 eggs. Scrambled
- 1 and 1/2 tablespoon coconut flour

How To

1. Preheat your oven to 350°F/175°C.
2. Mix the almond flour, salt, and baking powder in a bowl. Put to the side.
3. Add the butter and coconut oil to a skillet.
4. Melt for 20 seconds and pour into another bowl.
5. In this bowl, mix in the dough.
6. Scramble two eggs. Add to the dough.
7. Add 1/2 tablespoon of coconut flour to thicken, and place evenly into a cupcake tray. Fill about 3/4 inch.
8. Bake for 20 minutes until browned.
9. Allow to cool for 15 minutes and cut each in half for the buns.
10. Sandwich:
11. Fry the deli meat in a skillet on high heat.
12. Put the ham and cheese between the buns.
13. Heat the butter on medium-high.
14. When brown, turn too low and add the dough to the pan.
15. Press down with weight until you smell burning, then flip to crisp both sides.
16. Enjoy!

Nutrition (Per Serving)

- Calories: 230
- Fat: 21g
- Carbohydrates: 2g
- Protein: 15g

44.   Prosciutto Spinach Salad

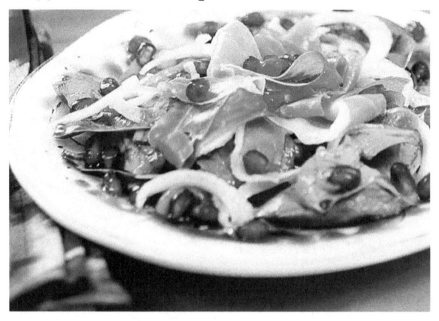

Serving: 4

Prep Time: 10 minutes

Cook Time: Ni

<u>Ingredients</u>

- 2 cups baby spinach
- 1/3 lb prosciutto
- 1 cantaloupe
- 1 avocado
- 1/4 cup diced red onion handful of raw, unsalted walnuts

How To

1. Put a cup of spinach on each plate.
2. Top with the diced prosciutto, cubes of balls of melon, slices of avocado, a handful of red onion, and a few walnuts.
3. Add some freshly ground pepper, if you like.
4. Serve!

Nutrition (Per Serving)

- Calories: 199
- Fat: 18g
- Carbohydrates: 2g
- Protein: 7g

Lasagna Spaghetti Squash

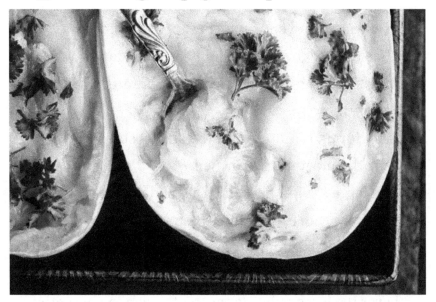

Serving: 4

Prep Time: 10 minutes

Cook Time: 60-80 minutes

Ingredients

- 25 slices mozzarella cheese
- 1 large jar (40 oz) Rao's Marinara sauce
- 30 oz whole-milk ricotta cheese
- 2 large spaghetti squash, cooked (44 oz)
- 4 lbs ground beef

How To

1. Preheat your oven to 375°F/190°C.
2. Slice the spaghetti squash and place it face down inside an oven-proof dish. Fill with water until covered.
3. Bake for 45 minutes until the skin is soft.
4. Sear the meat until browned.
5. In a large skillet, heat the browned meat and marinara sauce. Set aside when warm.
6. Scrape the flesh off the cooked squash to resemble strands of spaghetti.
7. Layer the lasagna in a large greased pan in alternating layers of spaghetti squash, meat sauce, mozzarella, ricotta. Repeat until all increases have been used.
8. Bake for another 30 minutes and serve!

Nutrition (Per Serving)

- Calories: 420
- Fat: 31g
- Carbohydrates: 5g
- Protein: 25g

46.   Blue Cheese Chicken Wedges

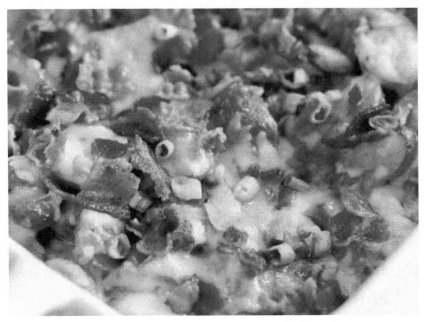

Serving: 4

Prep Time: 10 minutes

Cook Time: 30 minutes

Ingredients

- 2 tbsp crumbled blue cheese
- 4 strips of bacon
- 2 chicken breasts (boneless)
- 3/4 cup of your favorite buffalo sauce

How To

1. Boil a large pot of salted water.
2. Add two chicken breasts to the pot and cook for 28 minutes.
3. Turn off the heat and let the chicken rest for 10 minutes. Using a fork, pull the chicken apart into strips.
4. Cook and cool the bacon strips and put them to the side.
5. On medium heat, combine the chicken and buffalo sauce. Stir until hot.
6. Add the blue cheese and buffalo pulled chicken. Top with the cooked bacon crumbles.
7. Serve and enjoy.

Nutrition (Per Serving)

- Calories: 315
- Fat: 22g
- Carbohydrates: 8g
- Protein: 20g

47.   Feisty Bacon Snack

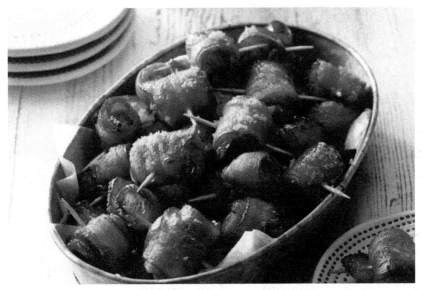

Serving: 4

Prep Time: 10 minutes

Cook Time: 60 minutes

Ingredients

- 30 slices thick-cut bacon
- 12 oz steak
- 10 oz beef sausage
- 4 oz cheddar cheese, shredded

How To

1. Lay out 5 x 6 slices of bacon in a woven pattern and bake at 400°F/200°C for 20 minutes until crisp.

2. Combine the steak, bacon, and sausage to form a meaty mixture.

3. Lay out the meat in a rectangle of similar size to the bacon strips. Season with salt/pepper.

4. Place the bacon weave on top of the meat mixture.

5. Place the cheese in the center of the bacon.

6. Roll the meat into a tight roll and refrigerate.

7. Make a 7 x 7 bacon weave and roll the bacon weave over the meat diagonally.

8. Bake at 400°F/200°C for 60 minutes or 165°F/75°C internally.

9. Let rest for 5 minutes before serving.

Nutrition (Per Serving)

- Calories: 388
- Fat: 38g
- Carbohydrates: 3g
- Protein: 29g

48.   Bacon And Scallops Snack

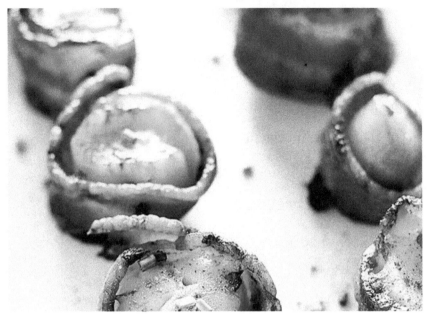

Serving: 4

Prep Time: 10 minutes

Cook Time: 6 minutes

<u>Ingredients</u>

- 12 scallops
- 12 thin bacon slices
- 12 toothpicks
- Salt and pepper to taste
- 1/2 tbsp oil

How To

1. Heat a skillet on high heat while drizzling in the oil.
2. Wrap each scallop with a piece of thinly cut bacon—secure with a toothpick.
3. Season to taste.
4. Cook for 3 minutes per side.
5. Serve!

Nutrition (Per Serving)

- Calories: 280
- Fat: 18g
- Carbohydrates: 3g
- Protein: 28g

49.   Perfect Gluten-Free Gratin

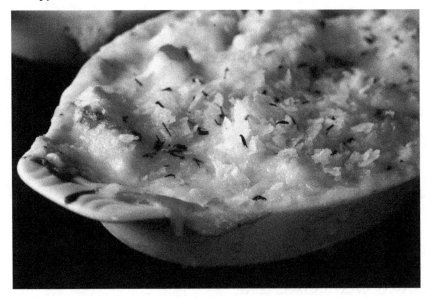

Serving: 4

Prep Time: 10 minutes

Cook Time: 20-25 minutes

Ingredients

- 4 cups raw cauliflower florets
- 4 tbsp butter
- 1 / 3 cup heavy whipping cream
- Salt and pepper to taste
- 5 deli slices pepper jack cheese

How To

1. Combine the cauliflower, butter, cream, salt, and pepper and microwave on medium for 20 minutes, or until tender.
2. Mash with a fork—season to your liking.
3. Lay the slices of cheese across the top of the cauliflower.
4. Cook inside your microwave for an additional 3 minutes, depending on the power of your microwave.
5. Serve!

Nutrition (Per Serving)

- Calories: 175
- Fat: 15g
- Carbohydrates: 3g
- Protein: 5g

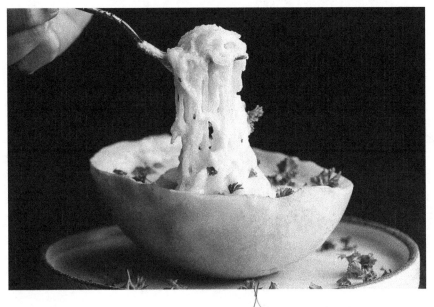

Serving: 4

Prep Time: 10 minutes

Cook Time: 25-30 minutes

Ingredients

- 1 tablespoon olive oil
- 1 and 1/2 pound sliced butternut squash
- Kosher salt & Black pepper
- 1 and 1/2 cup grated Parmesan cheese
- 2 oz. chopped bacon

How To

1. Set the oven to 4250F to preheat, then grease the baking tray
2. Add the olive oil in a medium skillet to heat to sauté the bacon, butternut squash, and the seasonings for 2 minutes.
3. After 2 minutes, pour everything on the baking tray to bake for 25 minutes
4. Remove from the oven, sprinkle the parmesan cheese on top the bake for 10 more minutes
5. Serve the meal while still warm.

Nutrition (Per Serving)

- Calories: 335
- Fat: 33g
- Carbohydrates: 12g
- Protein: 20g